ESSENTIAL GUIDE TO ACNE

Understanding, Treating, and Preventing Breakouts for Clearer Skin

DR. CASEY LOREN

DISCLAIMER

This book's content is only meant to be used for general informative purposes. Although the author has taken great care to ensure the content is accurate and thorough, no warranties or assurances on the information's accuracy, correctness, or reliability are provided. It is recommended that readers employ their own judgment and discretion when applying any material found in this book to their particular situation.

The information in this book is not intended to replace professional advice, nor is the author an expert in any of the subjects covered. It is recommended that readers consult with experienced professionals regarding any particular issues or concerns.

Any name that may be mentioned or referred in this book does not imply endorsement, recommendation, or relationship on the part of the author with any person, entity, good, website, or association. These references are made only for informational purposes and are not meant to be taken as recommendations or endorsements.

The information contained in this book may cause readers to suffer loss or damage, for which the author disclaims all obligation and accountability. The only people accountable for the decisions and actions taken by readers using the information presented are themselves.

Any names, characters, companies, locations, activities, occasions, and incidents referenced in this book are either made up or the result of the author's imagination. Any likeness to real people, living or dead, or to real things is entirely coincidental.

This book's content may change at any time, without prior notice, according to the author.

The onus is on the reader to verify whether there have been any updates or revisions.

The reader accepts the conditions of this disclaimer by reading this book. Please do not read this book or use its contents if you do not agree to these terms.

Table of Contents

CHAPTER 1

UNDERSTANDING ACNE

What is Acne?

Acne, often referred to as acne vulgaris, is a common skin condition characterized by the development of pimples, blackheads, whiteheads, and in severe cases, cysts or nodules. It typically affects areas rich in oil glands, such as the face, chest, back, and shoulders.

Types of Acne

Acne can manifest in various forms, including:

Whiteheads: Closed clogged pores filled with pus.

Blackheads: Open clogged pores with oxidized melanin.

Little red, swollen lumps called papules.

Pustules are red pimples that have pus at the ends.

Nodules: Large, painful, solid lesions beneath the skin.

Cysts: Deep, pus-filled, painful lesions.

Causes of Acne

Several factors contribute to acne development:

Excess Oil Production: Overactive sebaceous glands produce more oil, clogging pores.

Bacteria: Propionibacterium acnes (P. acnes) bacteria proliferate in clogged pores, leading to inflammation.

Hormonal Changes: Fluctuations in hormones, especially during puberty, menstruation, and pregnancy, can trigger acne.

Diet: Some studies suggest that high-glycemic diets or dairy consumption may exacerbate acne.

Genetics: A family history of acne can increase the likelihood of developing it.

Medications: Certain medications, like corticosteroids or hormonal treatments, may cause acne as a side effect.

Myths and Misconceptions about Acne

Common misconceptions about acne include:

Poor Hygiene Causes Acne: While hygiene is important, acne is primarily influenced by genetics, hormones, and other factors.

Acne is Just a Teenage Problem: Acne can affect people of all ages, from adolescence to adulthood.

Sun Exposure Clears Acne: While sun exposure may temporarily improve acne, it can worsen it in the long term and increase the risk of skin damage.

Popping Pimples Helps: Picking or popping pimples can lead to scarring, infection, and further inflammation.

Impact of Acne on Mental Health

Acne can significantly impact mental well-being:

Self-Esteem: Acne can lower self-esteem and confidence, leading to social anxiety and depression.

Psychological Distress: Severe acne may cause emotional distress, affecting daily life and relationships.

Body Image Concerns: Individuals with acne may experience body image issues and negative self-perception.

How Acne Develops

The development of acne involves several stages:

Increased Oil Production: Sebaceous glands produce excess oil (sebum).

Clogged Pores: Dead skin cells and oil-block hair follicles.

Bacterial Growth: P. acnes bacteria thrive in clogged pores.

Inflammation: Immune response causes redness, swelling, and pus formation.

Factors Contributing to Acne Development

Multiple factors influence acne development:

Hormonal Changes: Androgens stimulate oil production, contributing to acne during puberty and hormonal fluctuations.

Diet: High-glycemic foods and dairy products may exacerbate acne in susceptible individuals.

Stress: Emotional stress can worsen acne due to hormonal changes.

Medications: Certain medications, such as corticosteroids or hormonal treatments, can trigger or worsen acne.

Acne in Different Age Groups

Acne can affect individuals of all ages:

Adolescents: Common during puberty due to hormonal changes.

Adults: Acne can persist into adulthood or develop later due to hormonal imbalances, stress, or other factors.

Menopause: Hormonal shifts during menopause can trigger or worsen acne in some women.

Genetic Predisposition to Acne

Genetics play a significant role in acne development:

Family History: Individuals with a family history of acne are more likely to experience it themselves.

Genetic Variants: Certain genetic variations may influence sebum production, inflammation, and the skin's response to bacteria, impacting acne susceptibility.

Hormonal Influences on Acne

Hormones play a crucial role in acne development:

Androgens: Testosterone and other androgens stimulate sebaceous gland activity, leading to increased oil production and acne.

Estrogens: Estrogen levels influence sebum production and can affect acne severity.

Hormonal Fluctuations: Puberty, menstruation, pregnancy, and menopause are periods of hormonal changes that can trigger or exacerbate acne.

CHAPTER 2

SKIN ANATOMY AND PHYSIOLOGY

Overview of Skin Layers

The skin is the largest organ in the body and consists of three primary layers: the epidermis, dermis, and hypodermis (subcutaneous layer). The epidermis is the outermost layer, providing a protective barrier against pathogens, UV radiation, and water loss. Beneath the epidermis lies the dermis, which contains blood vessels, nerves, hair follicles, and glands. The hypodermis is primarily composed of fat cells that insulate the body and serve as an energy reserve.

Functions of the Skin

The skin performs various essential functions, including protection, sensation, temperature regulation, excretion, and vitamin D synthesis. Its protective barrier prevents pathogens from entering the body, while sensory receptors enable us to perceive touch, pressure, pain, and temperature. The skin also helps regulate body temperature through sweating and blood vessel dilation or constriction.

Knowledge of Sebaceous Glands

Sebaceous glands are microscopic glands located in the dermis that produce sebum, an oily substance that lubricates and waterproofs the skin and hair. Sebum helps maintain skin moisture and pH balance while also protecting against pathogens. However, the overproduction of sebum can contribute to acne formation.

Hair Follicles and Acne Formation

Tiny structures in the skin called hair follicles are where hair grows.

. Acne formation often occurs when hair follicles become clogged with excess sebum, dead skin cells, and bacteria. This leads to the development of comedones (blackheads and whiteheads), papules, pustules, nodules, or cysts, depending on the severity of the condition.

Role of Sweat Glands in Skin Health

Sweat glands, including eccrine and apocrine glands, play a crucial role in regulating body temperature and excreting waste products. Eccrine glands produce sweat that helps cool the body, while apocrine glands in areas like the armpits and groin produce thicker sweat that can contribute to body odor when mixed with bacteria.

The skin's pH balance is important for maintaining its protective barrier and overall health. The acidic pH of the skin (around 4.5-5.5) helps inhibit the growth of harmful bacteria and fungi. Disruptions in pH balance, often caused by factors like harsh skincare products or imbalances in sebum production, can contribute to acne development.

Importance of Collagen in Skin Integrity

The structural protein collagen gives the skin its flexibility and strength.

It plays a key role in maintaining skin integrity, firmness, and resilience. Factors such as aging, UV exposure, smoking, and poor nutrition can lead to collagen degradation, resulting in wrinkles, sagging, and reduced skin quality.

Skin's Natural Defense Mechanisms

The skin has several natural defense mechanisms to protect against pathogens and environmental damage. These include the acidic pH of the skin, the production of antimicrobial peptides, the shedding of dead skin cells, and the activation of immune responses when necessary.

Skin Regeneration Process

The skin has a remarkable ability to regenerate and repair itself. When injured, the body initiates a complex process involving inflammation, cell proliferation, and tissue remodeling. Skin regeneration is supported by factors such as adequate nutrition, hydration, and proper wound care.

Impact of External Factors on Skin Health

External factors such as UV radiation, pollution, smoking, diet, stress, and skin care products can significantly impact skin health. UV exposure, for example, can cause premature aging, and sunburn, and increase the risk of skin cancer. Pollution and toxins can contribute to inflammation and oxidative stress, leading to skin damage. Adopting a healthy lifestyle, protecting the skin from environmental stressors, and using appropriate skincare products are essential for maintaining optimal skin health.

Understanding these aspects of skin anatomy and physiology can provide valuable insights into maintaining healthy skin and managing conditions like acne effectively.

CHAPTER 3

PREVENTING ACNE SCARS AND HYPERPIGMENTATION

Early Intervention for Acne Scars:

Early intervention is key to preventing acne scars from forming. This involves promptly treating active acne to reduce inflammation and minimize the risk of scarring. Dermatologists recommend using over-the-counter or prescription medications containing ingredients like benzoyl peroxide, salicylic acid, or retinoids to control acne breakouts. Consulting with a dermatologist for personalized treatment is crucial, as they can recommend the most effective therapies based on individual skin types and acne severity.

Proper Wound Care to Prevent Scarring:

Proper wound care plays a vital role in preventing acne scars. It's essential to avoid picking, squeezing, or popping pimples, as this can worsen inflammation and lead to scarring. Instead, gently cleanse the skin with a mild cleanser and apply topical treatments recommended by a dermatologist. Keeping the skin hydrated and protected with a non-comedogenic moisturizer also aids in the healing process and reduces the likelihood of scarring.

Handling Hyperpigmentation After Inflammation (PIH):

Post-inflammatory hyperpigmentation (PIH) refers to dark spots or patches that occur after acne breakouts. Effective treatment options for PIH include topical retinoids, hydroquinone, azelaic acid, and vitamin C serums. These ingredients help fade pigmentation by promoting skin cell turnover and inhibiting melanin production. Sun protection is crucial when treating PIH to prevent further darkening of pigmented areas.

Sun Protection for Preventing Hyperpigmentation:

Sun protection is paramount in preventing hyperpigmentation, including PIH and melasma. UV exposure can worsen existing pigmentation and hinder the effectiveness of treatments. Using a broad-spectrum sunscreen with SPF 30 or higher daily, seeking shade during peak sun hours, wearing protective clothing, and using hats or sunglasses can help minimize sun-induced pigmentation and protect overall skin health.

Importance of Gentle Skincare in Scar Prevention:

Gentle skincare practices are essential for scar prevention, especially for individuals prone to acne. Harsh products and aggressive cleansing can irritate the skin, exacerbate inflammation, and delay healing. Opting for gentle, non-abrasive cleansers, avoiding scrubbing or over-exfoliating, and using soothing ingredients like aloe vera or chamomile can promote skin health and minimize the risk of scarring.

Avoiding Picking and Squeezing Pimples:

Avoiding the urge to pick or squeeze pimples is crucial in preventing acne scars. Manipulating acne lesions can lead to further inflammation, rupture of the follicle wall, and subsequent scarring. Instead, practicing hands-off skincare, using spot treatments containing benzoyl peroxide or salicylic acid, and applying non-comedogenic moisturizers can help manage acne without causing additional damage to the skin.

Professional Treatments for Scar Prevention:

Dermatological interventions offer effective solutions for scar prevention and treatment. Dermal fillers, chemical peels, microneedling, and laser therapy are available options.

These treatments target acne scars by stimulating collagen production, resurfacing the skin, and improving overall texture. Consulting with a board-certified dermatologist or skincare professional is recommended to determine the most suitable treatment plan based on individual skin concerns and scar types.

Managing Acne to Minimize Scarring Risk:

Properly managing acne is essential for minimizing the risk of scarring. This includes adopting a consistent skincare routine, avoiding pore-clogging products, and identifying triggers that exacerbate breakouts. Dermatologists may recommend oral medications, such as antibiotics or isotretinoin, for severe or persistent acne cases. Combining medical treatments with lifestyle modifications, such as a balanced diet and stress management, can significantly reduce acne-related scarring.

Addressing Hyperpigmentation in Different Skin Types:

Hyperpigmentation can affect individuals with various skin types, requiring tailored treatment approaches. People with darker skin tones are more prone to developing PIH and may benefit from ingredients like niacinamide, kojic acid, or licorice extract to address pigmentation concerns. It's essential to consult with a dermatologist familiar with diverse skin types to ensure safe and effective treatment options that minimize the risk of post-inflammatory pigmentation.

Long-Term Strategies for Scar Prevention:

Long-term scar prevention strategies involve ongoing skincare maintenance and lifestyle adjustments. Consistently using sunscreen, practicing gentle skincare habits, and avoiding environmental factors that trigger acne breakouts or pigmentation are key components. Additionally, regular follow-ups with a dermatologist for acne management and scar assessment can help monitor progress and make necessary adjustments to treatment plans. Adopting a holistic approach to skincare and wellness promotes long-lasting results in scar prevention.

CHAPTER 4

LIFESTYLE AND ACNE MANAGEMENT

Importance of Diet in Acne Management

Diet plays a crucial role in managing acne. While individual responses can vary, certain dietary patterns have been associated with acne flare-ups. Foods with a high glycemic index, such as sugary snacks and refined carbohydrates, can spike blood sugar levels, leading to increased oil production and inflammation in the skin, potentially worsening acne. On the other hand, a diet rich in antioxidants, vitamins, and minerals from fruits, vegetables, whole grains, and lean proteins can support skin health and reduce acne severity. It's also essential to stay hydrated as dehydration can affect skin barrier function and exacerbate acne symptoms.

Hydration and Its Impact on Skin Health

Hydration is paramount for overall skin health, including acne management. Adequate water intake helps maintain skin hydration, supports the skin's natural barrier function, and aids in flushing out toxins that can contribute to acne. However, excessive washing or using harsh products can strip the skin of its natural oils, leading to dryness and potential irritation, which can aggravate acne. Opt for gentle cleansers and moisturizers suitable for acne-prone skin to maintain a healthy moisture balance.

Sleep and Stress Management Techniques

Quality sleep is vital for skin repair and overall well-being. Lack of sleep can disrupt hormonal balance, increase stress levels, and contribute to inflammation, all of which can worsen acne. Incorporating stress management techniques such as mindfulness, meditation, yoga, or deep breathing exercises can help reduce stress hormones like cortisol, which can impact sebum production and acne development. Establishing a regular sleep schedule and creating a relaxing bedtime routine can also promote better sleep quality.

Exercise and Its Influence on Acne

Regular exercise offers numerous benefits for overall health, including potential benefits for acne management. Physical activity improves blood circulation, reduces stress, and supports hormonal balance, all of which can positively impact skin health. However, excessive sweating during workouts can lead to clogged pores if not properly cleansed afterward, so it's essential to cleanse the skin gently post-exercise and avoid tight-fitting clothing that can trap sweat and bacteria against the skin.

Skincare Routine for Acne-Prone Skin

A tailored skincare routine is crucial for managing acne-prone skin. Start with a gentle cleanser suitable for acne, followed by an oil-free moisturizer to maintain hydration without clogging pores. Incorporate acne-fighting ingredients such as salicylic acid or benzoyl peroxide in your routine, but introduce them gradually to avoid irritation. Use non-comedogenic (non-pore-clogging) products and avoid excessive scrubbing or picking at acne lesions to prevent further inflammation and scarring.

Choosing the Right Cosmetics for Acne

When selecting cosmetics for acne-prone skin, opt for oil-free, non-comedogenic formulas labeled as "acne-safe" or "suitable for acne-prone skin." Look for products that won't clog pores or exacerbate acne, such as mineral-based makeup and non-greasy sunscreens. Avoid heavy, pore-clogging products like thick foundations or creams, and remember to remove makeup thoroughly before bed to prevent pore blockages and breakouts.

Sun Protection and Acne

While sunlight can temporarily improve acne due to its drying effect, excessive sun exposure can lead to skin damage and worsen acne in the long run. Use a non-comedogenic sunscreen with at least SPF 30 daily, even on cloudy days or indoors, to protect your skin from harmful UV rays. Choose lightweight, oil-free sunscreens specifically designed for acne-prone skin to avoid pore blockages.

Smoking and Acne Connection

Smoking can have detrimental effects on skin health, including acne. Smoking contributes to oxidative stress, impairs blood flow, and damages collagen, all of which can exacerbate acne and delay healing. Quitting smoking can significantly improve overall skin condition, including acne severity, and promote better skin health in the long term.

Alcohol and Acne: What You Need to Know

Alcohol consumption, particularly heavy drinking, can impact skin health and contribute to acne development. Alcohol can dehydrate the skin, leading to increased oil production to compensate, potentially clogging pores and triggering breakouts. Moreover, alcohol consumption can disrupt hormonal balance and compromise the skin's natural barrier function, making it more susceptible to acne. Moderation or avoiding alcohol altogether can benefit both overall health and acne management.

Managing Acne Flare-Ups

Despite preventive measures, acne flare-ups can still occur. It's essential to have a plan for managing flare-ups effectively. Avoid picking or squeezing acne lesions as it can worsen inflammation and lead to scarring. Instead, use spot treatments with acne-fighting ingredients like benzoyl peroxide or salicylic acid to target individual breakouts. Maintain a consistent skincare routine, manage stress levels, and consider consulting a dermatologist for personalized treatment options such as prescription medications or professional procedures if needed.

By addressing these aspects comprehensively, individuals can develop a holistic approach to acne management that encompasses lifestyle factors, skincare routines, and informed choices for overall skin health.

CHAPTER 5

PSYCHOLOGICAL IMPACT OF ACNE

1. Acne and Self-Esteem: Acne can significantly affect an individual's self-esteem. Visible acne lesions may lead to feelings of embarrassment, shame, and lowered self-confidence. The perception of one's appearance can play a crucial role in self-esteem, especially during adolescence and young adulthood when peer comparisons are common. It's essential to address these feelings by focusing on inner qualities, and achievements, and seeking effective acne management strategies.

2. Coping Strategies for Acne-Related Stress: Managing stress related to acne involves adopting healthy coping mechanisms. These may include practicing mindfulness and relaxation techniques, maintaining a balanced lifestyle with proper nutrition and exercise, engaging in hobbies and activities that bring joy, and seeking professional support if stress becomes overwhelming.

3. **Social Anxiety and Acne:** Acne can contribute to social anxiety, where individuals may feel anxious or self-conscious in social situations due to their appearance. Cognitive-behavioral strategies, such as challenging negative thoughts and gradual exposure to social settings, can be beneficial. Developing social skills and building self-acceptance also play vital roles in managing social anxiety related to acne.

4. **Depression and Acne:** The link between acne and depression is well-documented. Chronic acne can lead to feelings of sadness, hopelessness, and a lack of interest in activities. It's crucial to recognize the signs of depression and seek professional help when needed. Treatment options may include therapy,

medication, and lifestyle changes to improve mental well-being.

5. Body Dysmorphic Disorder (BDD) and Acne: Some individuals with acne may develop Body Dysmorphic Disorder (BDD), a condition characterized by obsessive preoccupation with perceived flaws in appearance. Treatment often involves therapy, such as cognitive-behavioral therapy (CBT), to address distorted beliefs and improve body image perception.

6. Impact of Acne on Relationships: Acne can impact relationships, including romantic relationships and friendships. Communication, empathy, and understanding are key in navigating these challenges. Open discussions about feelings and concerns related to acne can strengthen relationships and foster support.

7. Seeking Professional Help for Emotional Support: When dealing with the emotional impact of acne, seeking professional help is crucial. Psychologists, counselors, and dermatologists can provide support, guidance, and treatment options tailored to individual needs.

8. Building Confidence While Managing Acne: Building confidence involves focusing on personal strengths, setting realistic goals, and practicing self-care. Emphasizing inner qualities and achievements can boost self-esteem and confidence, even while managing acne.

9. Peer Support Groups for Acne Sufferers: Joining peer support groups for acne sufferers can provide a sense of belonging, shared experiences, and emotional support. These groups can offer valuable insights, coping strategies, and encouragement in dealing with the challenges of acne.

10. Holistic Approaches to Mental Wellness: Taking a holistic approach to mental wellness involves addressing physical, emotional, and social aspects of well-being. This may include practicing self-compassion, engaging in activities that promote relaxation and joy, fostering supportive relationships, and seeking professional guidance when needed.

By understanding and addressing the psychological impact of acne through these various perspectives and strategies, individuals can work towards improved mental well-being and a more positive outlook despite the challenges posed by acne.

CHAPTER 6

NATURAL REMEDIES FOR ACNE

Tea Tree Oil: Benefits and Application

Tea tree oil has gained recognition for its potent anti-inflammatory and antimicrobial properties, making it a popular natural remedy for acne. It contains compounds like terpinen-4-ol that help reduce inflammation and combat acne-causing bacteria, such as Propionibacterium acnes.

When using tea tree oil for acne, it's crucial to dilute it with a carrier oil like coconut oil or jojoba oil to prevent skin irritation. A general recommendation is to mix one part of tea tree oil with nine parts of the carrier oil before applying it to the affected areas using a cotton swab.

Aloe Vera for Acne Treatment

Aloe vera is renowned for its soothing and healing properties, making it an excellent choice for acne-prone skin. It contains compounds like aloin and gibberellin that possess anti-inflammatory and wound-healing effects, aiding in the reduction of acne redness and swelling.

To use aloe vera for acne, extract the gel from a fresh aloe vera leaf and apply it directly to the affected areas. Leave it on for about 10-15 minutes before rinsing off with lukewarm water. Regular use can help improve acne symptoms and promote clearer skin.

Honey and Cinnamon Mask

The combination of honey and cinnamon is a popular home remedy for acne due to its antibacterial and anti-inflammatory properties. Honey contains enzymes that help unclog pores and reduce inflammation, while cinnamon has antimicrobial properties that can combat acne-causing bacteria.

To make a honey and cinnamon mask, mix equal parts of raw honey and cinnamon powder to form a paste. Apply the mask to clean skin and leave it on for 10-15 minutes before rinsing off with warm water. This mask can help soothe acne-prone skin and promote a clearer complexion over time.

Zinc Supplements for Acne

Zinc is an essential mineral that plays a crucial role in skin health and immune function. It is known for its anti-inflammatory and antioxidant properties, making it beneficial for managing acne. Zinc helps regulate sebum production, reduce inflammation, and support the healing of acne lesions.

Taking zinc supplements as part of an acne treatment plan can be beneficial, especially for individuals with zinc deficiency or hormonal acne. However, it's essential to consult a healthcare professional for the correct dosage and duration of supplementation to avoid potential side effects.

Green Tea Extracts and Acne

Green tea extracts are rich in antioxidants called catechins, particularly epigallocatechin gallate (EGCG), which exhibit anti-inflammatory and antimicrobial properties. These compounds help reduce inflammation, regulate sebum production, and inhibit the growth of acne-causing bacteria.

Using skincare products containing green tea extracts or applying cooled green tea as a toner can benefit acne-prone skin. Additionally, drinking green tea regularly can provide internal antioxidant support, contributing to overall skin health and acne management.

Witch Hazel is a Natural Astringent

Witch hazel is a natural astringent derived from the witch hazel shrub. It has astringent properties that help tighten pores, reduce excess oil production, and soothe inflammation, making it a popular choice for acne-prone skin.

To use witch hazel for acne, apply it to clean skin using a cotton ball or pad as a toner. Avoid using witch hazel products that contain alcohol, as they can be drying and irritating to the skin. Opt for alcohol-free witch hazel preparations for best results.

Essential Oils for Acne Prone Skin

Certain essential oils like lavender, rosemary, and chamomile possess anti-inflammatory, antimicrobial, and soothing properties that can benefit acne-prone skin. These oils help reduce inflammation, fight acne-causing bacteria, and promote a calmer complexion.

When using essential oils for acne, it's crucial to dilute them with a carrier oil to avoid skin irritation. Popular carrier oils include jojoba oil, coconut oil, and almond oil. Conduct a patch test before applying diluted essential oils to larger areas of the skin to check for sensitivity.

Apple Cider Vinegar for Acne

Apple cider vinegar (ACV) has antimicrobial and exfoliating properties that make it a popular natural remedy for acne. It contains acetic acid, which helps regulate skin pH, reduce bacteria growth, and unclog pores, leading to clearer skin.

To use ACV for acne, dilute it with water in a 1:3 ratio (one part ACV to three parts water) and apply it to the skin using a cotton pad as a toner. It's essential to patch test first and gradually increase the ACV concentration if tolerated well. Avoid using undiluted ACV directly on the skin, as it can irritate.

Dietary Supplements for Acne Management

Certain dietary supplements can support acne management by addressing underlying factors such as inflammation, hormonal imbalance, and oxidative stress. Supplements like omega-3 fatty acids, probiotics, vitamin A, and zinc have shown promise in improving acne symptoms.

Before starting any dietary supplements for acne, consult a healthcare professional to determine the appropriate dosage and suitability based on individual needs. Supplements should complement a healthy diet and skincare routine, not replace them entirely.

Herbal Remedies for Acne

Several herbal remedies have been traditionally used to treat acne due to their anti-inflammatory, antibacterial, and skin-soothing properties. Herbs like neem, turmeric, licorice root, and calendula can help reduce acne symptoms and promote clearer skin.

Herbal remedies for acne can be used topically in the form of creams, serums, or masks, or taken internally as supplements or herbal teas. It's essential to research each herb's benefits, potential side effects, and interactions before use, especially if combining multiple herbal remedies. Consulting a healthcare professional or herbalist can provide personalized guidance.

CHAPTER 7

DEALING WITH ACNE IN SPECIFIC POPULATIONS

Acne in Adolescents: Common Challenges

Acne in adolescents is a prevalent concern due to hormonal changes during puberty, which trigger increased oil production and clogged pores. These changes often lead to blackheads, whiteheads, and inflamed pimples. The emotional impact can be significant, affecting self-esteem and social interactions. Treatment typically involves gentle skin care, topical treatments like benzoyl peroxide or retinoids, and sometimes oral medications for severe cases.

Acne in Adults: Causes and Treatment Approaches

Adult acne can stem from hormonal fluctuations, stress, genetics, or lifestyle factors like diet and skincare habits. Treatment strategies focus on addressing the underlying cause while minimizing irritation. Topical retinoids, salicylic acid, and oral medications such as antibiotics or hormonal therapies may be prescribed. Lifestyle changes like stress management and a balanced diet can also play a crucial role.

Acne in Pregnancy: Safety Concerns

Managing acne during pregnancy requires special consideration due to the potential risks associated with certain medications. Pregnant individuals are advised to avoid retinoids, tetracycline antibiotics, and hormonal therapies like spironolactone. Instead, they can opt for gentle cleansers, topical azelaic acid, or glycolic acid under medical supervision to ensure safety for both mother and baby.

Acne in Men: Skincare Tips

Men often experience acne due to excess oil production, shaving irritation, or hormonal imbalances. Skincare tips for men include using non-comedogenic products, gentle cleansing after shaving, and incorporating exfoliation with salicylic acid or glycolic acid. Maintaining a consistent routine and avoiding harsh products can help manage breakouts effectively.

Acne in Women: Hormonal Influences

Hormonal fluctuations throughout the menstrual cycle can trigger acne in women. Managing hormonal acne may involve birth control pills, spironolactone, or topical treatments like hormonal creams or retinoids. Tailoring skincare routines to the menstrual cycle phases and addressing underlying hormonal imbalances are key strategies for women dealing with acne.

Acne in People of Color: Unique Considerations

People of color may experience post-inflammatory hyperpigmentation (PIH) more prominently after acne lesions heal. This requires a tailored approach to prevent and treat PIH, including avoiding harsh treatments, using sunscreen daily, and incorporating skin-lightening agents like azelaic acid or kojic acid under dermatological guidance.

Acne in Elderly Individuals

While acne is commonly associated with youth, elderly individuals can also experience late-onset acne due to hormonal changes or medication side effects. Treatment may involve gentle cleansers, topical retinoids, or oral medications based on the individual's health status and skin sensitivity. Regular skin care routines and periodic dermatological evaluations are essential for managing acne in older adults.

Acne in Athletes: Managing Sweat-Induced Breakouts

Athletes often face acne triggered by sweat, heat, and friction from equipment or clothing. Prevention involves wearing breathable fabrics, showering promptly after workouts, and using non-comedogenic skincare products. Exfoliation with salicylic acid can help unclog pores and reduce breakouts associated with sweat-induced acne.

Acne in Patients with Chronic Illnesses

Patients with chronic illnesses may experience acne due to medication side effects, hormonal imbalances, or stress. It's crucial to consult healthcare providers for acne management tailored to the individual's medical condition and medication regimen. Gentle skincare, topical treatments, and lifestyle adjustments can help alleviate acne symptoms without exacerbating underlying health issues.

Acne in LGBTQ+ Community: Addressing Specific Needs

Members of the LGBTQ+ community may face unique challenges related to acne, including hormonal changes from gender-affirming therapies or stress from societal factors. Healthcare providers should offer inclusive and understanding care, considering the individual's medical history, gender identity, and specific skincare needs. Collaboration between patients and healthcare professionals can lead to effective acne management and improved overall well-being.

CHAPTER 8

MEDICAL TREATMENTS FOR ACNE

Over-the-Counter (OTC) Acne Products:

Over-the-counter (OTC) acne products are a first-line treatment for many individuals dealing with mild to moderate acne. They are accessible without a prescription and come in various forms such as creams, gels, cleansers, and spot treatments. These products typically contain active ingredients like benzoyl peroxide, salicylic acid, sulfur, or resorcinol. They work by targeting the causes of acne, such as excess oil production, inflammation, and bacterial growth.

When using OTC acne products, it's crucial to follow the instructions carefully and be patient as results may take several weeks to become noticeable. Some people may experience mild irritation or dryness initially, but these side effects often improve with continued use. If you don't see improvement after a few weeks or if your acne is severe, it's advisable to consult a dermatologist for further evaluation and treatment.

Topical Treatments: Retinoids, Benzoyl Peroxide, and Salicylic Acid:

Topical treatments are a cornerstone of acne management and can be obtained both over the counter and through prescription.

Retinoids: These are derivatives of vitamin A and work by unclogging pores, promoting cell turnover, and reducing inflammation. Common retinoids include adapalene, tretinoin, and tazarotene. They are available in various strengths and formulations, such as creams, gels, and lotions.

Benzoyl Peroxide: Benzoyl peroxide is an antibacterial agent that helps kill acne-causing bacteria and reduces excess oil production. It is available in different concentrations and can be found in cleansers, creams, and spot treatments.

Salicylic Acid: Salicylic acid exfoliates the skin, unclogs pores, and reduces inflammation. It is often found in acne washes, toners, and spot treatments.

These topical treatments may cause some initial dryness, redness, or peeling, especially during the first few weeks of use. Gradually introducing them into your skincare routine and using a moisturizer can help minimize these side effects.

Oral Medications for Acne:

In some cases, oral medications may be prescribed to treat acne, particularly if it is moderate to severe or resistant to topical treatments. Common oral medications for acne include antibiotics, hormonal therapies, and isotretinoin.

Antibiotics: Oral antibiotics such as doxycycline, minocycline, and tetracycline are often prescribed to reduce acne-causing bacteria and inflammation. They are usually used for a limited period to avoid antibiotic resistance.

Hormonal Therapy for Acne in Women: Hormonal fluctuations can contribute to acne, especially in women. Hormonal therapies such as birth control pills containing estrogen and progestin or anti-androgen medications may be recommended to help regulate hormone levels and improve acne.

Isotretinoin (Accutane) for Severe Acne: Isotretinoin is a powerful oral medication reserved for severe, nodular acne that hasn't responded to other treatments. It works by reducing oil production, shrinking oil glands, and preventing acne formation. However, it comes with potential side effects and requires close monitoring by a healthcare provider.

Light Therapy for Acne:

Light therapy, also known as phototherapy, is a non-invasive treatment that uses different wavelengths of light to target acne-causing bacteria, reduce inflammation, and promote skin healing. Common types of light therapy for acne include blue light therapy, red light therapy, and a combination of both (photodynamic therapy). Light therapy is typically performed in a dermatologist's office and may require multiple sessions for optimal results.

Chemical Peels and Microdermabrasion:

Chemical peels and microdermabrasion are cosmetic procedures that can help improve acne and acne scars by exfoliating the outer layer of the skin and promoting cell turnover.

Chemical Peels: Chemical peels involve applying a chemical solution to the skin, which causes the outer layer to peel off, revealing smoother, rejuvenated skin underneath. They can help reduce acne, improve skin texture, and diminish the appearance of acne scars.

Microdermabrasion: Microdermabrasion uses a handheld device to exfoliate the skin and remove dead skin cells. It can help unclog pores, reduce blackheads and whiteheads, and improve overall skin tone and texture.

These procedures are usually performed by trained professionals and may require multiple sessions to achieve the desired results. It's important to follow post-procedure care instructions and protect the skin from sun exposure.

Injectable Treatments for Acne Scars:

Injectable treatments such as dermal fillers and corticosteroid injections can be used to improve the appearance of acne scars.

Dermal Fillers: Dermal fillers containing hyaluronic acid or other substances can help fill in depressed acne scars and improve skin texture.

Corticosteroid Injections: Corticosteroid injections are used to reduce inflammation and flatten raised or hypertrophic acne scars. They are typically administered by a dermatologist and may require multiple treatments for optimal results.

These injectable treatments can provide temporary or long-lasting improvements in acne scars, depending on the type of treatment used and the individual's skin response.

Combination Therapies for Stubborn Acne:

For stubborn or severe acne that doesn't respond well to single treatments, combination therapies may be recommended. This approach involves using multiple treatments simultaneously or sequentially to target different aspects of acne, such as inflammation, bacterial growth, and excess oil production. For example, a combination of topical retinoids, benzoyl peroxide, and oral antibiotics may be prescribed to address different acne-related factors and improve overall outcomes. Dermatologists tailor combination therapies based on the individual's skin type, severity of acne, and treatment goals. Regular follow-ups and adjustments to the treatment plan may be necessary to achieve and maintain clear skin.

Understanding the range of medical treatments available for acne and working closely with a dermatologist can help individuals find effective solutions tailored to their unique needs and preferences.

CHAPTER 9

PREVENTING ACNE SCARS AND HYPERPIGMENTATION

Early Intervention for Acne Scars:

Early intervention is crucial in preventing acne scars from forming. When acne lesions are still active, they can cause inflammation and damage to the skin, leading to scarring. Dermatologists often recommend starting treatment as soon as acne appears to minimize the risk of scarring.

Proper Wound Care to Prevent Scarring:

Proper wound care is essential in preventing scars from forming after acne lesions heal. This includes keeping the affected area clean, avoiding picking or squeezing pimples, and using gentle skincare products to promote healing without causing further irritation.

Handling Hyperpigmentation After Inflammation (PIH):

Post-inflammatory hyperpigmentation (PIH) is a common concern after acne breakouts. It manifests as dark spots or patches on the skin and can take weeks or even months to fade. Treatment options include topical products containing ingredients like vitamin C, niacinamide, and hydroquinone, as well as procedures like chemical peels and laser therapy.

Sun Protection for Preventing Hyperpigmentation:

Sun protection is crucial in preventing hyperpigmentation, including PIH, from worsening. UV rays can darken existing pigmentation and prolong the healing process. Daily use of sunscreen with a high SPF, wearing protective clothing, and avoiding peak sun hours can help prevent hyperpigmentation.

Importance of Gentle Skincare in Scar Prevention:

Gentle skincare is key in scar prevention, especially for acne-prone skin. Harsh products can irritate the skin, exacerbate acne, and lead to more significant scarring. Opt for non-comedogenic and fragrance-free products that are gentle yet effective in maintaining skin health.

Avoiding Picking and Squeezing Pimples:

Picking and squeezing pimples can worsen inflammation, increase the risk of infection, and lead to more severe scarring. It's essential to resist the urge to pick at acne lesions and instead focus on proper skincare and treatment under the guidance of a dermatologist.

Professional Treatments for Scar Prevention:

Dermatologists offer various professional treatments to prevent and reduce acne scars. These include laser therapy, microneedling, chemical peels, and dermal fillers. These treatments target different types of scars and can significantly improve the skin's appearance.

Managing Acne to Minimize Scarring Risk:

Effective acne management is critical in minimizing the risk of scarring. This may involve topical or oral medications, lifestyle changes, and skincare routines tailored to the individual's skin type and severity of acne. Consulting with a dermatologist can help develop a personalized acne management plan.

Addressing Hyperpigmentation in Different Skin Types:

Hyperpigmentation can affect different skin types differently, requiring tailored treatment approaches. Darker skin tones are more prone to PIH and may benefit from ingredients like azelaic acid and kojic acid, while lighter skin tones may respond well to hydroquinone and retinoids. Dermatologists can recommend suitable treatments based on skin type and pigmentation concerns.

Long-Term Strategies for Scar Prevention:

Long-term scar prevention involves consistent skincare habits, regular dermatologist visits for monitoring and treatment adjustments, and lifestyle choices that promote skin health. This includes maintaining a balanced diet, staying hydrated, managing stress, and avoiding habits like smoking that can impair skin healing.

By implementing these strategies and seeking professional guidance when needed, individuals can effectively prevent acne scars and hyperpigmentation, promoting clearer and healthier skin over time.

CHAPTER 10

ACHIEVING CLEAR SKIN AND MAINTAINING RESULTS

Setting Realistic Expectations for Acne Treatment

Understanding that acne treatment is a gradual process is key. Expecting immediate results can lead to disappointment and frustration. It's crucial to realize that each person's skin is unique, and what works quickly for one person may take longer for another. Professional guidance can help set realistic timelines and goals based on individual skin types and conditions.

Patience and Consistency in Skincare Routines

Consistency is the cornerstone of effective skincare. Establishing a routine that includes gentle cleansing, appropriate acne treatments, moisturizing, and sun protection is essential. Patience is equally important; skin changes often take weeks or even months to become noticeable. It's about staying committed to the routine and trusting the process.

Tracking Progress and Adjusting Treatments

Keeping track of skin changes, both positive and negative, is vital. This can involve taking photos regularly or maintaining a journal to note any shifts in acne severity or skin health. Based on these observations, adjustments to skincare products or treatment plans may be necessary.

Consulting with a dermatologist ensures these adjustments are informed and beneficial.

Recognizing Improvements in Acne

Sometimes, improvements in acne can be subtle. Understanding what constitutes progress beyond just clear skin, such as reduced inflammation, fewer breakouts, or improved texture, is important. Acknowledging these smaller victories can motivate you to continue with the skincare regimen.

Transitioning from the Treatment to the Maintenance Phase

As acne improves, transitioning from intensive treatment to a maintenance phase is a natural progression. This phase focuses on sustaining clear skin while adjusting the skincare routine accordingly. It may involve fewer active acne-fighting ingredients and more emphasis on hydration and protection.

Importance of Follow-Up Visits with Dermatologists

Regular follow-up visits with a dermatologist are crucial for ongoing acne management. These appointments allow for monitoring progress, discussing any concerns or changes in skincare needs, and receiving professional guidance on long-term maintenance strategies. Dermatologists can also address any new skin issues that may arise.

Lifestyle Changes for Long-Term Acne Management

Incorporating healthy lifestyle habits can complement acne treatment and contribute to long-term skin health. This includes maintaining a balanced diet, staying hydrated, managing stress levels, getting enough sleep, and avoiding triggers like excessive sun exposure or harsh skincare products.

Embracing Skin Health as a Journey

Viewing skin health as a journey rather than a quick fix reframes the mindset around acne management. It acknowledges that achieving and maintaining clear skin requires ongoing effort, patience, and adaptability. Embracing this perspective fosters a positive relationship with skincare and overall well-being.

Confidence Building Exercises

Building confidence goes hand in hand with clear skin. Engaging in self-care practices, such as positive affirmations, mindfulness exercises, or activities that bring joy and fulfillment, can boost self-esteem. Confidence is about feeling comfortable in one's skin, regardless of imperfections.

Celebrating Clear Skin Achievements

Finally, celebrating milestones and achievements in clear skin is important. Whether it's reaching a specific skincare goal, noticing significant improvements, or simply feeling more confident, acknowledging these victories reinforces positive behaviors and motivates continued dedication to skincare routines.

By integrating these aspects into an essential guide to acne, individuals can navigate their acne journey with patience, understanding, and empowerment.